YAKALOU MEDIA

ARE YOU READY FOR A BABY TODAY?

Let's Find Out With These 100 Insightful "Yes Or No" Questions

Contents

Disclaimer

This book is designed to provide information only. This information is provided and sold with the knowledge that the publisher and author do not offer any legal or other professional advice. In the case of a need for any such expertise, consult with the appropriate professional.

This book does not contain all the information available on the subject. This book has not been created to be specific to any individual's or organization's situation or needs. Every effort has been made to make this book as accurate as possible. However, there may be typographical and/or content errors. Therefore, this book should serve only as a general guide, not as the ultimate source of subject information.

This book contains information that might be dated and is intended only to educate and entertain. Regarding any loss or damage allegedly suffered or alleged to have occurred as a result of the information in this book, either directly or indirectly, the author and publisher shall have no liability or responsibility to any person or entity.

I

Part One

Introduction

Welcome to "Are You Ready For A Baby?" If you've picked up this book, you're likely pondering that very question. This journey of introspection and self-discovery we're about to embark on together is no small feat. In fact, it's one of the most significant explorations you can undertake in your life. But don't worry—we're here to navigate this path together, through clarity and simplicity, one thoughtful question at a time.

Why this book, you might ask? Let's consider this: bringing a new life into the world is a profound decision, impacting not only you but also the life you'll be shaping and guiding. It goes beyond biological readiness; it's about emotional, financial, lifestyle, and personal readiness. It's about understanding the essence of parenthood. Yet, how often do we dive deep into these aspects before deciding to become parents? That's where this book steps in.

You see, this book isn't just a guide—it's your companion. With it, we aim to create a space for introspection and a platform to evaluate your readiness across different facets of your life. We use straightforward, everyday language, breaking down complex considerations into comprehensible parts. The objective is not to intimidate but to enlighten, not to deter but to prepare.

At the heart of this book are 100 deep and thought-provoking

Yes or No questions spread across 10 pivotal categories, each dedicated to an essential aspect of readiness. From understanding yourself and evaluating your relationship to considering your financial stability, career trajectory, emotional preparedness, and more, these questions are designed to make you pause and ponder, to elicit honest reflections and insights.

Perhaps you'll find some questions straightforward, while others may provoke deeper contemplation. Some answers may affirm your readiness, while others may highlight areas needing further consideration. But that's the beauty of this journey—it's tailored to your unique experiences, aspirations, and circumstances. And remember, it's not a test—it's a tool for self-awareness and preparation.

As we embark on this enlightening journey, keep an open mind, be honest with yourself, and remember, this isn't about reaching a definitive 'yes' or 'no'. It's about understanding, preparing, and making informed decisions. So, are you ready to delve deep, to uncover, and to discover? Are you ready to ask yourself, "Am I ready to have kids today?" Let's find out together.

What Will You Learn in This Book

As we journey further, it's vital to clarify what you can expect and caution against potential misconceptions. This chapter aims to set the right expectations while alerting you to the inherent limitations that come with a tool like this.

Let's begin with the lessons you'll uncover in this book. At its core, this book is a guide to self-discovery and readiness evaluation. Through 100 thought-provoking Yes or No questions, you'll explore various aspects of your life that contribute to your readiness for parenthood.

You'll assess your understanding of yourself, your relationship, your financial situation, career considerations, emotional readiness, health and lifestyle, social support, your living situation, your future goals, and your understanding of parenthood.

Each chapter is an invitation to dive deep into these categories, unraveling the layers of considerations, expectations, and realities tied to each one. By answering these questions honestly, you'll gain insights into your readiness and areas that might need more attention or discussion.

However, a word of warning is necessary here. While this book is a tool designed to help you reflect, it isn't a predictor or a decision-maker. The insights gained should serve as starting points for further thought, discussion, and possibly professional consultation. This book doesn't offer absolute answers because parenthood, like life, isn't about absolutes. It's complex, personal, and unique to each individual and couple.

Remember, a 'Yes' or 'No' response to any question isn't a final verdict on your readiness. It's simply an indicator of where you stand at this moment. It's okay, and completely normal, to have mixed feelings or uncertainties. It's okay to move between 'Yes' and 'No' as you progress in your journey.

Another point of caution: this book shouldn't replace professional advice. If you're struggling with certain aspects, such as health or financial concerns, consider reaching out to professionals in these fields. They can provide advice tailored to your unique circumstances and needs.

In conclusion, this book will guide you to explore and evaluate your readiness for parenthood. It'll illuminate areas of strength and highlight areas needing further reflection or action. But remember, it's a guide—not a magic ball. It's here to help you ask the right questions, not to hand over definite answers.

So, embark on this journey with an open mind, knowing that each question is a step toward understanding yourself better and making an informed decision about becoming a parent. Are you ready to take that step?

The "Yes or No Questions" Concept

With the groundwork laid, it's time to dive into the fun part of our journey: the Yes or No questions. But before we embark, let's spend some time understanding the "Yes or No Questions Concept". Why yes or no? What's the idea behind this approach? In this chapter, we'll delve into these queries, setting the stage for the enlightening journey ahead.

Imagine standing at a crossroad with multiple paths branching out. It's confusing, isn't it? Which one should I choose? Where does each lead? Now, picture the same crossroad, but with just two paths - Yes or No. It's simpler, clearer, and less daunting, right? That's the beauty of the Yes or No approach. It simplifies the complex process of self-evaluation, offering a clear starting point for your reflections.

This simplicity, however, doesn't mean that these questions lack depth. On the contrary, each question is designed to provoke thought, stirring up reflections on various aspects of your life. When you answer 'Yes' or 'No', you're not just responding to the question at face value; you're exploring the thoughts, feelings, and experiences that led you to that answer.

Here's where it gets interesting: Your answers may surprise you. You might find some questions easier to respond to than others, and some answers are more certain than others. This variance, this mix of certainty and uncertainty, is where the real insights lie. It's a reflection of your readiness, your values, and your aspirations—all crucial factors in assessing your preparedness for parenthood.

Now, a word of caution: while the Yes or No approach simplifies things, it doesn't mean your journey ends at the answer. Consider each response as a doorway to deeper reflection. Ask yourself, 'Why did I answer yes or no? What experiences or beliefs influenced my answer? What does this say about my readiness?'

In this journey of self-discovery, the questions are your roadmap, the Yes or No responses your compass, guiding you through the terrain of your thoughts, feelings, and experiences. Together, they'll aid you in navigating this complex, enriching journey toward understanding your readiness for parenthood.

As we move forward into the heart of this book, remember: each Yes or No isn't a conclusion; it's an invitation to dive deeper, to reflect, to understand. So, are you ready to explore these yeses and nos, to uncover the insights they hold? Let's embark on this journey together.

The Rules Of The "Yes or No" Questions

Are you ready for the next step in our journey? Great! Let's delve into the "Yes or No Questions" game concept. But wait, a game with rules? Absolutely! Even though it's more of an introspective exploration than a traditional game, having some guidelines will help you navigate this process more effectively. So let's lay down the rules for our game of self-discovery and readiness evaluation.

Rule 1: Honesty Is Key. The first rule is as simple as it gets, yet it's the most crucial one. Be honest with your answers. Remember, the purpose here isn't to get all 'Yes' answers but to reflect truthfully on each question. Only through sincere responses can you truly gauge your readiness and uncover deeper insights.

Rule 2: There Are No Right or Wrong Answers. This isn't a test you pass or fail. Each question is designed to provoke thought, not to score points. Your 'Yes' or 'No' isn't about right or wrong; it's about what feels right for you, given your experiences, values, and aspirations.

Rule 3: Pause and Reflect. Don't rush through the questions.

Take your time to consider each one fully and to delve into the feelings and thoughts it stirs up. The value isn't just in the final 'Yes' or 'No'; it's in the journey to that answer.

Rule 4: Keep an Open Mind. Some questions might challenge your beliefs or make you uncomfortable. That's okay. Approach them with an open mind and a willingness to explore different perspectives. You might be surprised by what you discover about yourself.

Rule 5: Revisit and Revise. Your answers might change over time, and that's completely fine. Feel free to revisit the questions as your circumstances, feelings, or perspectives change. This book is designed to be a companion on your journey, not a one-time exercise.

Finally, a word to remember: this "game" isn't about winning or losing. It's about self-discovery, readiness evaluation, and thoughtful preparation for one of life's most significant decisions: becoming a parent. It's about asking yourself tough questions, reflecting on your values and circumstances, and learning about your strengths and areas for growth.

Are you ready to play the game by these rules? Are you ready to embark on this enlightening journey of self-discovery and readiness evaluation? Let's dive into the "Yes or No Questions" game together.

II

100 Insightful Yes or No Questions

Chapter 1: Understanding Yourself

It's no small feat to think about bringing a new life into this world. It requires a lot of introspection, understanding, and readiness. We've chosen this chapter to be the first one, as self-evaluation is always the starting point. It's essential to acknowledge and analyze your thoughts, feelings, and abilities before proceeding. Remember, honesty is your best friend here.

Before you start dreaming about baby names and nursery decorations, it's important to pause and ask yourself: "Am I ready to be a parent?" Let's dive into the deep end of introspection, shall we? This journey may challenge you, but it will also clarify your thoughts. You need to assess your feelings about starting a family and gauge if you are mentally, emotionally, and physically ready to have a child.

This chapter can also serve as a foundation to evaluate your relationship with your partner. Having children is a shared responsibility that requires mutual agreement, a shared vision, and consistent cooperation. Are you and your partner both on the same page about having children? Your answer could significantly impact your decision. It's necessary to ensure that both partners are equally enthusiastic about welcoming a new member into your family.

Now, let's get started. Here are 10 Yes or No questions designed to help you evaluate your readiness. Reflect on these questions honestly, and remember, there are no wrong answers, only insights.

1. Are you happy with the person you are today?
2. Do you feel emotionally stable and content most of the time?
3. Are you willing to change your lifestyle for a child?
4. Do you feel ready to take on the responsibility of another human being's life?
5. Are you comfortable discussing your feelings, thoughts, and worries with your partner?
6. Do you and your partner communicate effectively about important decisions?
7. Are you and your partner equally enthusiastic about starting a family?
8. Can you easily resolve conflicts with your partner and reach a mutual agreement?
9. Do you feel your relationship with your partner is strong and stable?
10. Are you willing to prioritize the needs of a child above your own?

These questions are your stepping stones to understanding yourself better and evaluating your readiness to have a child. This process is not about rushing or pushing yourself; instead, it's about being honest and understanding your feelings. After all, you're considering a life-changing decision. So take your time, and remember, it's okay to have doubts or fears. They're part of the process.

As you proceed, always keep in mind that it's not just about being ready for a baby; it's about being ready to become a parent. Now, let's move forward on this journey of self-discovery. Happy introspecting!

Chapter 2: Relationship Evaluation

After journeying through the self, it's now time to shift our lens to your relationship. Because having children is not just a solitary decision—it's a joint venture, an extension of the bond you share with your partner. This chapter invites you to deeply assess the strength, resilience, and harmony in your relationship.

In the course of parenthood, your relationship will be tested and stretched in ways you've never imagined. It's a profound commitment that transcends just the two of you. You and your partner will need to navigate sleepless nights, disagreements over parenting styles, financial stresses, and more. Understanding your relationship dynamics and how you operate as a team under stress is a key aspect of preparing for parenthood.

As you delve into this chapter, remember that no relationship is perfect. Each one is unique, woven with its own strengths and imperfections. It's normal to have disagreements and face challenges. What's critical is how you handle those disagreements, how you communicate, and how you find resolutions together.

The following 10 Yes or No questions are designed to help you gauge the health of your relationship. As you read each one, take a moment to reflect. Be open, be honest, and remember, there's no right or wrong—only growth.

1. Do you feel that your relationship with your partner is balanced and equal?
2. Are you satisfied with the level of communication in your relationship?
3. Do you feel your relationship could withstand the stresses of having a child?
4. Can you discuss difficult topics with your partner without leading to a heated argument?
5. Do you feel supported and loved by your partner?
6. Are you and your partner able to bounce back from arguments and disagreements positively?
7. Do you trust your partner implicitly, and do you believe they trust you just as deeply?
8. Does your partner respect your opinions and decisions?
9. Are you comfortable with the level of emotional intimacy in your relationship?
10. Do you see your partner as a good future parent?

Reflect on these questions, but don't rush. This is a process of understanding and coming to grips with where you and your partner stand. It's perfectly alright to identify areas that might need work. It's better to address them now than let them become points of tension later.

And remember, this journey of evaluation is not about judging your relationship; it's about fortifying it. You're preparing to welcome a new life into your world—a commitment that's all the more beautiful when it's shared and nurtured in a strong, loving relationship. Onward we journey, deeper into the heart of readiness.

Chapter 3: Financial Preparation

Now that we've explored self-awareness and relationship dynamics, let's dive into a different but crucial aspect of preparation: your finances. In this chapter, we will delve into the economic side of things. It might not sound as emotional or deep as the previous two chapters, but trust us, it is just as critical.

Having children is a joy like no other, but let's be realistic—it also comes with significant financial responsibilities. From diapers to education, raising a child requires a considerable amount of financial resources. It's not about having enough money to provide the most lavish lifestyle, but about being prepared for the necessities and the unexpected.

While money should never be a determining factor in your decision to have children, financial stability can indeed make the journey less stressful. It allows you to focus on the joys of parenting without constant worry about meeting basic needs. Therefore, being proactive about your financial planning is a step you can't afford to skip.

We've prepared a set of 10 Yes or No questions to guide you through this important aspect of your readiness evaluation. As always, honesty is key. There's no perfect score—only an opportunity for understanding and planning.

1. Do you have a stable source of income?
2. Have you built an emergency fund that can cover unexpected expenses?
3. Are you comfortable with your current lifestyle expenses?
4. Do you feel prepared for additional costs like childcare, healthcare, and education for a child?
5. Have you considered the financial impact of a potential parental leave from work?
6. Are you financially ready to make changes to your home to accommodate a child?
7. Do you have a clear understanding of your insurance needs for a future child?
8. Are you willing to adjust your spending habits to meet your child's needs?
9. Can you financially support a child even if unexpected expenses arise?
10. Have you started considering long-term financial planning for your child's future?

It's normal if these questions stir a bit of worry or uncertainty. Finances can feel overwhelming, but remember, the goal here is not to frighten but to prepare. The journey to financial readiness is not a sprint; it's a marathon. Take your time, make a plan, and be patient with yourself.

As we close this chapter, we want to emphasize that financial readiness isn't about wealth—it's about planning and preparation. It's about having the foresight to meet the beautiful challenge of parenthood with prudence and confidence. And with that, let's step forward to our next chapter on the path to readiness.

Chapter 4: Career Considerations

Now that we've scrutinized our finances, let's turn our attention to another significant part of our lives—our careers. In this chapter, we'll consider how the decision to have children could impact your professional life. Because, let's face it, balancing a career and parenting is like walking a tightrope—sensational, challenging, and requiring careful consideration.

Our careers are not just about earning a livelihood. They're often closely tied to our identities, ambitions, and self-esteem. Yet, when children enter the picture, your professional life might need to adapt. There could be changes in working hours, possible career breaks, the need for childcare, and more.

Importantly, this chapter isn't intended to deter you, but to prepare you. It's about understanding the possible changes that having a child might bring to your career path and ensuring that you're ready to manage them. It's about ensuring that you can provide for your child, not just materially but also with time, care, and presence.

So, take a deep breath and prepare yourself for another set of Yes or No questions designed to shed light on your career preparedness. Remember, there are no right or wrong answers, only meaningful reflections.

1. Do you feel secure in your current job?
2. If needed, can your job provide flexibility for parental duties?
3. Are you aware of your company's parental leave policies?
4. Have you considered the impact of possible career breaks or reduced working hours?
5. If your job demands frequent travel, are you ready to modify these commitments?
6. Are you prepared for the possibility that parenting duties may occasionally disrupt your work routine?
7. Have you considered the costs and logistics of childcare during working hours?
8. Do you and your partner have a plan to share parental responsibilities to manage career demands?
9. Can you handle work stress and parental responsibilities simultaneously?
10. Are you willing to put career advancements on hold, if required, for your child's needs?

Reflecting on these questions will help you understand your career readiness when contemplating parenthood. Remember, it's okay if your answers reveal that you have more work to do. Identifying these areas gives you the chance to plan, adapt, and make the necessary arrangements.

And as we close this chapter, remember this: Parenthood is about balance. While careers are important, they are only one facet of our lives. Just as you commit to your work, commit to the journey of parenthood.

With planning and adaptability, you can find a harmonious balance that supports both your family and your professional aspirations. As you embark on this path, we hope you find strength, resilience, and joy. Let's stride ahead toward the next chapter of readiness.

Chapter 5: Emotional Readiness

Having journeyed through understanding yourself, evaluating your relationship, assessing your financial situation, and contemplating your career, let's now delve into your emotional preparedness. This chapter is all about introspecting on your emotional health, resilience, and readiness for the joys and challenges of parenting.

Becoming a parent isn't just about practical preparations and arrangements. It's a profound emotional commitment. Parenthood brings an array of emotions, from overwhelming love to high stress, immense joy to bouts of anxiety. It's a roller-coaster ride, and you need to ensure your emotional wellbeing is prepared for it.

Emotional readiness involves understanding your capacity to handle stress, your ability to provide emotional support to a child, and your willingness to prioritize the needs of your family. It's about being resilient in the face of sleepless nights, temper tantrums, and the constant worries that come with parenting.

We've crafted a set of 10 Yes or No questions to help you reflect on your emotional readiness. As always, honesty is crucial. Take your time, ponder each question, and remember: it's all part of your preparation journey.

1. Are you emotionally stable most of the time?
2. Can you handle high-stress situations without becoming overwhelmed?
3. Do you feel you have the emotional capacity to provide constant care and support to a child?
4. Are you comfortable expressing and managing your emotions?
5. Are you ready to put your child's emotional needs above your own when necessary?
6. Can you remain patient and understanding in the face of challenging child behaviors?
7. Do you have a strong support system to turn to during emotionally difficult times?
8. Are you ready to handle the anxiety and worry that comes with parenting?
9. Can you handle the emotional changes that might come with having a child?
10. Do you feel emotionally mature enough to guide a child through their own emotional growth?

These questions are intended to guide you toward a better understanding of your emotional readiness to become a parent. It's perfectly okay if you find areas where you might need a bit more preparation. Identifying these areas is the first step toward strengthening your emotional resilience.

Remember, emotional readiness is not about perfection. It's about understanding and strengthening your emotional well-being for yourself and your future family. The journey to emotional readiness is not a sprint; it's a journey of continuous growth and learning. And with each step, you're becoming more prepared for the beautiful challenge that is parenthood. Let's continue moving forward on our path to readiness.

Chapter 6: Health and Lifestyle

As we continue our journey to evaluate readiness for parenthood, we now turn our focus to a fundamental aspect of your preparation—your health and lifestyle. This chapter encourages you to assess the physical, nutritional, and lifestyle factors that play a pivotal role in the parenthood journey.

Raising a child is physically demanding and requires a certain level of health and stamina. It's not just about being ready to chase after a toddler or carry a growing baby; it's about having the energy to be present and engaged in your child's life. Moreover, your lifestyle choices—such as nutrition, exercise, sleep, and work-life balance—can significantly influence your ability to handle the demands of parenthood.

The decision to become a parent might also require you to make certain lifestyle changes. You might need to reconsider habits like late-night social events, spontaneous travel, or even simple things like uninterrupted sleep or personal time. This does not imply that your life will become less exciting or joyful, only that it might change as a result of the rewards and obligations of parenthood.

Let's dive into the next set of 10 Yes or No questions. They're designed to guide your reflections on health and lifestyle readiness. As you navigate through these, remember to be honest with yourself. There are no right or wrong answers, just valuable insights.

1. Do you consider yourself to be in good health?
2. Are you prepared to handle the physical demands of pregnancy or adoption processes?
3. Are you ready to commit to a healthy lifestyle for the well-being of your child?
4. Have you considered how a child will impact your current sleep patterns?
5. Can you incorporate regular exercise into your routine to maintain good health?
6. Are you prepared to provide nutritious meals for your family?
7. Can you handle the changes in your social life that might come with parenthood?
8. Do you understand the health responsibilities associated with raising a child?
9. Are you ready to prioritize your health and well-being to be a present and capable parent?
10. Are you willing to adapt your current lifestyle to cater to a child's needs?

Reflecting on these questions will help you understand your readiness to make health and lifestyle adjustments for parenthood. It's alright if some answers highlight areas that need work. Identifying these areas gives you the opportunity to make changes and improvements.

Remember, becoming a parent doesn't mean abandoning who you are or the lifestyle you enjoy. It's about adapting, growing, and integrating your child into your life's journey. With preparation and flexibility, you can build a healthy, balanced life for yourself and your family. Now, let's continue this exciting journey of readiness.

Chapter 7: Social Support

As we delve further into your readiness journey, we now turn to an often overlooked yet vital aspect of preparation: your social support system. This chapter is designed to help you assess the presence and strength of your support networks and their role in your journey to parenthood.

Parenting, while rewarding and fulfilling, can sometimes feel like a challenging solo expedition. That's where your social support system comes in. It can consist of family, friends, neighbors, community groups, or professional networks. These supportive individuals and groups can provide emotional comfort, practical help, valuable advice, or just a friendly ear when you need to vent.

Having a strong social support system can make the transition to parenthood smoother and more enjoyable. It doesn't mean you're not capable of handling things on your own, but rather acknowledges that having others to lean on can make the journey less overwhelming and more manageable.

So, let's examine your social support through another set of 10 Yes or No questions. Remember, these questions are for reflection and introspection, so honesty is key.

1. Do you have family or friends who support your decision to have children?
2. Is there someone in your life who can provide practical assistance when needed (such as babysitting or helping with household tasks)?
3. Do you have someone you trust to talk to about your doubts, fears, or anxieties related to parenthood?
4. Are you comfortable asking for help when you need it?
5. Do you feel a sense of support from your neighborhood or community?
6. Do you have access to professional resources (like pediatricians, psychologists, or support groups) for parenting advice?
7. Are you willing to expand your social network to include other parents or parent groups?
8. Do you feel you can rely on your partner for emotional and practical support?
9. Are you prepared to support your partner's emotional and practical needs?
10. Do you have people in your life who can step in during emergencies or times of high stress?

Reflecting on these questions will provide insights into your social support readiness. If you find areas that need improvement, take it as an opportunity to build stronger connections and networks.

Remember, seeking and accepting support is not a sign of weakness; it's a testament to the community spirit that has defined human survival and progress. As we close this chapter, know that no parent is an island, and it's okay to lean on others.

Embrace your social support, for it will not only lighten your load but also enrich your journey toward parenthood. Let's continue our exploration in the next chapter of readiness.

Chapter 8: Living Situation

This chapter nudges you to evaluate your current living conditions and their suitability for a new addition. Our surroundings impact us significantly, and for a child, their home environment can greatly influence their growth, safety, and sense of security.

Whether it's the physical space, the neighborhood, proximity to schools, or access to parks and recreational facilities, all these factors are essential when considering a child. Perhaps your current home is a bustling city apartment, a suburban house, or a countryside cottage; each of these presents unique opportunities and challenges when raising a child.

Additionally, your living situation also includes the people you live with. If you're living with extended family or roommates, how will having a child affect these dynamics? Alternatively, if it's just you and your partner, are you prepared for the changes a baby will bring?

Let's explore these considerations through our next set of 10 Yes or No questions. As you answer them, think about your current living situation and how it might need to change or adapt.

1. Do you have enough space in your home to comfortably accommodate a child?

2. Is your living environment safe and secure for a child?
3. Do you have access to child-friendly amenities like parks or recreational facilities?
4. Are there suitable educational institutions like schools and daycare centers nearby?
5. If you live with others, are they supportive and prepared for the changes a baby will bring?
6. If you need to move for more space or a better environment, are you financially prepared for that?
7. Are you ready to adapt your living space to be child-friendly (like baby-proofing)?
8. Is your neighborhood conducive to raising a child?
9. Are you prepared to handle the household chores that will increase with a child?
10. Do you have a plan for managing late-night feedings, early wake-up calls, and other child-related disruptions to your living routine?

Reflecting on these questions will help you assess whether your current living situation is conducive to bringing a child into the world and what changes you might need to make. Identifying areas that need improvement is an opportunity to plan and prepare.

Remember, every home is unique, and there's no perfect living situation. It's about creating a loving, secure, and stimulating environment that nurtures your child's development.

As we close this chapter, know that homes are made with love and adaptability, and it's this love that turns a living space into a welcoming nest for your child. Let's carry these reflections forward to the next chapter of our readiness journey.

Chapter 9: Future Goals and Plans

As you progress on your readiness journey, it's time to take a broad view and consider how a child fits into your long-term goals and plans. This chapter invites you to consider your aspirations and how parenthood might influence and shape them.

Life doesn't pause with parenthood, and neither do your personal and professional aspirations. It's essential to think about how a child would fit into your plans, whether they involve career growth, further education, travel, retirement, or anything else. It's about finding the balance between pursuing your dreams and providing a stable, nurturing environment for your child.

Also, consider what you envision for your child's future. What kind of education and opportunities would you want for them? How do you plan to support them as they grow and develop their own dreams and goals?

Let's delve into these long-term considerations with the next set of 10 Yes or No questions. Take your time with these, for they demand a glimpse into your future.

1. Have you considered how a child will fit into your long-

term personal goals?

2. Have you thought about how parenthood might impact your career plans?
3. If you have plans for further education, have you considered how a child would fit into this?
4. Do you have a plan for balancing your personal interests and hobbies with the demands of parenthood?
5. If you have aspirations to travel, have you thought about how a child might influence these plans?
6. Are you willing to make adjustments to your long-term plans to accommodate the needs of a child?
7. Have you considered your child's future education and opportunities?
8. Are you ready to support your child as they develop their own dreams and goals?
9. Do you have a plan for managing your retirement while providing for your child's needs?
10. Have you and your partner discussed and aligned your future goals regarding parenthood?

Reflecting on these questions will give you a clearer vision of your future and how a child can be a part of it. If you find some areas need further consideration, embrace it as a chance to plan and strategize better.

Remember, adding a child to your long-term plans doesn't mean giving up on your dreams. It's about integrating your aspirations with your responsibilities as a parent.

As we move toward the last chapter of our readiness journey, carry with you the understanding that dreams and parenthood can coexist beautifully, shaping a future filled with growth and love.

Chapter 10: Understanding of Parenthood

Welcome to the final chapter, "Understanding of Parenthood". Having assessed various facets of your life in the preceding chapters, we now delve into the essence of this journey—understanding what parenthood truly entails. This chapter aims to help you reflect on your comprehension of what being a parent means, beyond the physical, financial, and practical aspects.

Parenthood isn't just about providing for a child's needs; it's about nurturing, guiding, teaching, and learning. It's about being there for the first steps, the first words, the school plays, the soccer matches, and even the teenage heartbreaks. But it's also about managing tantrums, dealing with sleepless nights, making tough decisions, and often putting your child's needs above your own.

An understanding of parenthood is also about acknowledging its uncertainties. No matter how much you prepare, unexpected things can and will happen. It's about being flexible and patient, learning on the go, and forgiving yourself when you make mistakes.

Let's explore your understanding of parenthood through our final set of 10 Yes or No questions. As always, honesty is paramount as you reflect on these points.

1. Do you understand that parenthood involves more than just providing for a child's basic needs?
2. Are you prepared for the emotional challenges that parenthood can bring?
3. Do you understand that parenthood requires constant learning and adaptation?
4. Are you ready to put your child's needs above your own when necessary?
5. Do you acknowledge that every child is unique and may not meet conventional expectations?
6. Are you prepared for the responsibility of guiding and teaching a child?
7. Do you understand that parenting is a lifelong commitment?
8. Are you ready to face and manage the uncertainties that parenthood may present?
9. Can you forgive yourself and learn from your mistakes as a parent?
10. Are you ready to experience the joys, challenges, love, and learning that comes with parenthood?

Reflecting on these questions will help you understand your perceptions of parenthood and where they might need refinement. It's okay if you don't have all the answers; parenthood is a journey of continuous growth and learning.

As we conclude this chapter and the book, remember that readiness for parenthood isn't about perfection. It's about willingness—the willingness to change, to learn, to love, to be patient, and to prioritize another human being.

If this book has helped you on your journey of reflection and preparation, then it has served its purpose. As you step forward into the world of parenthood or decide to wait a bit longer, know that you are wiser and better prepared for having taken this introspective journey.

How To Interpret The Results

Welcome to this insightful chapter, where we guide you in understanding what your answers mean. Now that you've journeyed through each chapter, reflecting deeply on your circumstances, aspirations, and understanding of parenthood, it's time to make sense of your responses. This chapter will help you interpret your results, but remember, this process is less about the final score and more about the introspection you've experienced along the way.

So, you've answered a total of 100 questions, a thorough checklist that spans various aspects of your life. You've been honest and thoughtful, which is commendable. Now, let's take a look at the number of 'Yes' responses you've given.

If you've answered 'Yes' to 80 or more questions, that's a strong indication that you're well-prepared for the journey of parenthood. Your readiness spans personal understanding, relationship stability, financial security, career compatibility, emotional preparedness, health considerations, social support, suitable living situations, future plans, and a deep understanding of parenthood. This doesn't mean you'll have no challenges or doubts, but it shows you've considered many vital aspects and feel confident to take the next step.

What if your 'Yes' answers fall between 50 and 79? Well, this suggests you're on your way but may have a few areas to think more about or work on. Parenthood is a big decision, and it's essential to feel ready in all aspects of your life. Review the chapters where your 'No' responses were dominant. Do these areas require more time, resources, or discussions with your partner?

If you've answered 'Yes' to fewer than 50 questions, it seems like there are quite a few areas you're unsure about, and that's okay. Parenthood is a life-changing decision, and it's crucial to take all the time you need to feel ready. It might be beneficial to revisit certain chapters, do some additional research, or have conversations with parents you know.

Remember, these interpretations are not a strict pass-or-fail grade. They're here to guide you, providing a clearer understanding of your readiness for parenthood based on your current life circumstances. No test can definitively tell you if you're ready to be a parent. That decision is deeply personal and unique to every individual and couple.

Take your time, digest the results, and think about your next steps. Whether you're ready to embrace parenthood, need more time to prepare, or decide to explore a different path, remember that this journey of introspection and self-discovery you've embarked upon is invaluable.

It's made you pause and think, assess and reassess, dream and plan—proving that no matter what, you are ready to make thoughtful and responsible decisions about your life.

This brings us to the end of our guide. We hope this introspective journey has been insightful and helpful, providing you with clarity and confidence as you navigate the exciting landscape of potential parenthood.

What Is Your Result?

What is your result?

How many Yes or No answers do you have?

Yes =

No =

Are You Ready For A Baby?

Are You Ready For A Baby?

Your Answer:

What are your thoughts?

Conclusion: Taking The Next Steps Together

And here we are, at the end of our journey together, but perhaps just the beginning of your personal journey toward understanding your readiness for parenthood. You've dug deep, reflected, learned, and grown through this process, and for that, I commend you. It takes courage to ask ourselves tough questions, to face our truths, and to be open to self-discovery, and you've done just that.

I want to take this moment to thank you. Thank you for trusting this book to be a part of your journey. Thank you for your willingness to explore, to question, and to reflect. Your courage and openness are what make this book meaningful, and for that, I am deeply grateful.

As we part ways, remember that your journey doesn't end with this book. The questions we've explored and the insights you've gained are stepping stones to guide you on your path toward making the best decision for you and your family.

Now, I have a humble request. If you found this book helpful in your journey, could you please leave a review? Your feedback not only helps me understand how to better serve readers like you, but it also helps others who might be standing at the precipice of this significant life decision. Your words could be the beacon of light that guides them toward this tool, allowing them to gain the same insights and clarity that you've found.

Remember, each review has the power to reach someone, to resonate with them, and to assure them they're not alone in their thoughts, fears, and aspirations. Your experience and your voice could be the helping hand they need in their journey. So, I kindly ask you to take a few moments to leave a review. Share your experience, your thoughts, and your learnings. You never know whose life you might touch with your words.

Once again, thank you for accompanying me on this journey and for investing your time and trust in this book. I hope it has been a valuable companion in your journey toward understanding your readiness for parenthood. As you move forward, I wish you courage, clarity, and joy in all that you choose to do. Your journey is unique, and however you choose to navigate it, remember that you're not alone. We're in this together. Thank you, and take care.

www.ingramcontent.com/pod-product-compliance
Lightning Source LLC
Chambersburg PA
CBHW060845260726

48661CB00002B/627